Primal Diet Made Easy:

Lose Weight, Get More Energy and Improve Your Overall Health

By

Brittany Samons

Table of Contents

Primal Diet Made Easy: Lose Weight, Get More Energy and Improve Your Overall Health

By Brittany Samons

Introduction

The Primal diet is an advanced food arrangement focused around the assumed eating methodology of ancient cave people. It is focused on a phrase "if a cave man didn't consume it, you shouldn't consume it". Since heredity have changed little since the beginning of horticulture, advanced people are adjusted to the eating regimen or weight control plans of the Primal period.

The eating methodology commonly comprises of fish, grass-bolstered eggs, vegetables, pasture-raised meats, apples and oranges, parasites, roots, and nuts, and avoids what are seen to be farming items: grains, vegetables, dairy items, refined salt, potatoes, handled oils and refined sugar. It is contended that human populaces subsisting today on weight control plans thought to be like that of our Primal progenitors are generally free of illnesses of prosperity.

Chapter 1. Purpose of Primal Diet

For weight reduction, the Primal diet, which is the thing that our ancestors consumed when they needed to chase or accumulate their nourishment as opposed to developing it, would appear to be a decent thought. It's high in protein and fiber—and any individual who's ever attempted to shed pounds has been advised that the privileged insights to thinning down are protein and fiber, which take more time to travel down the digestive framework making us feel more full more. Prepared sugars, then again, hurdle through our framework making us hungry seemingly minutes after we've put down the fork

The high-fiber part, Primal diet aficionados keep up, is the key. Since fiber is bulkier and harder to method, it is a desire preparation by with success turning off appetite signs. But that is not what researchers discovered when they put the antiquated Primal eat less carbs under serious scrutiny in a test tube. The sort of grasses our predecessors consumed hold insoluble filaments that the body doesn't break down much, so they may not trigger ravenousness smothering indicators of different sorts of fiber. That doesn't mean insoluble fiber isn't beneficial for you; it is. It's what's in verdant greens, some apples and oranges, and loads of vegetables. In any case it doesn't send your cerebrum the satiety indicates the way dissolvable fiber does. Dissolvable fiber, nonetheless, is metabolized by the body to create intensifies that set off the indicator to the cerebrum that the body has had enough.

Primal diet is a life-style that includes attempting to consume and practice in the same way that our Primal progenitors did keeping in mind the end goal to enhance your physical fitness. Individuals who have picked along these lines of consuming are reporting that they lose fat easily and that they just need to do an hour or two of activity a week with a specific end goal to get fit as a fiddle. The thinking behind the primal method for living is that the human genome has changed. However we now consume a totally distinctive eating regimen that our body has not adjusted to. This is the reason more individuals are overweight or fat, even kids less than 10 years of age are getting fat. The data that individuals are getting from the legislature and nutritionists is definitely not acting as many individuals' battle to shed pounds through decreasing their fat admission or by attempting to consume less. Consuming in a primal or style is truly simple. You simply wipe out everything that came after the agrarian revolution. This methods vegetables like peanuts, grain items like bread and rice and in addition potatoes. It goes without saying that all prepared nourishment is out of the image. As an alternative you must eat meat, crunchy vegetables and tree grown foods, eggs, fish and nuts. In the event that you take a gander at the sorts of sustenance that we ought to dispense with and think you perceive a theme that numerous individuals have unfavorably susceptible responses to them then you are correct. Numerous individuals are lactose and gluten bigoted, more proof that we didn't advance to have the capacity to consume those parts.

It's staggeringly simple to get more fit succeeding this eating methodology in light of the fact that your body no more changes over all the sugar and carbs into fat. While in the meantime you feel full in view of the protein you are consuming. You additionally don't generally need to measure shares in view of this. The issue with all the sugar, starches and salt is that they make you feel much hungrier and thirstier, you never feel fulfilled by consuming those sorts of transformed nourishments. The primal diet of lean meat and nature's unmodified abundance can support, and even recuperate human science. The primal eating methodology reinforces what the present day eating regimen devastates. The primal eating methodology cuts human physiology down to the right weight and with less fat in the body and better nourishment in the sustenance, the slimmer human body is more effective and sound, other than being more trim and excellent. Several individuals have discovered a more young weight and body style, and additionally new life from this primal eating regimen of products of the soil, nuts, characteristic vegetation and lean meat. Primal diet formulas are basic and scrumptious, simple to make and to eat. Not just is the sustenance less handled before being sold to people in general, it needs less preparing in the kitchen before it is consumed. It's less work for more weight reduction and more prominent wellness, an inside and out champ.

Chapter 2. Recommended and Prohibited Foods

Basically, Primal lifestyle and eating methodology take motivation and signals from our progenitors and the way we used to consume and live. It's not about re-authorizing the Stone Age time yet rather it's powered by advanced experimental and restorative exploration and practical judgment skills.

The eating methodology concentrates on natural, entire nourishments, heaps of sound fats including soaked fat, grass-encouraged, unfenced meat and eggs, bunches of fish and fish, vegetables, soil grown foods, berries, nuts, seeds and some characteristic sweeteners. It avoids grains, vegetables, handled sugar and generally dairy. Some incorporate solid dairy nourishments like kefir, full fat regular yogurt, and some matured cheddar and spread obviously – it truly relies on upon your sensitivities. I cherish thusly of consuming in light of the fact that it additionally centered on nearby, natural produce and great cultivating practices.

The primal lifestyle additionally pushes healthier resting propensities, stress decrease, practical wellness, sufficient sun presentation, staying away from ecological poisons etc.

Most importantly, primal is not a situated of strict guidelines, it's to a greater degree a system that you can adjust focused around your own particular objectives, wellbeing, sex, age, area and current lifestyle. It's an extremely comprehensive methodology to health.

Recommended Foods

Meat and poultry (counting offal) – grass-encouraged, unfenced meat is not just a kinder and more moral approach to devour creature items yet it is additionally much higher in supplements due to the way the dairy cattle was sustained and raised.

Fish and fish – attempt to pick manageable, wild fish and fish when conceivable

Eggs – unfenced, pasture raised at whatever point conceivable

Vegetables – non-starchy and starchy tubers and root vegetables

Leafy foods – stick to low sugar products of the soil and keep high sugar apples and oranges like bananas and mangos for a considerable length of time when you require a higher carbs allow or when in season and tasting tasty.

Nuts and seeds – these gentlemen are nutritious yet numerous nuts and seeds are high in Omega-6 unsaturated fats which might be expert incendiary if expended in extensive amounts and when you're eating regimen is not offset by an equivalent measure of Omega-3 unsaturated fats found in slick fish like salmon and sardines, eggs and verdant greens. Fundamentally, don't glut on containers of nuts and seeds consistently. The same strives for nut suppers and flours, for example, almond feast.

Flavors and herbs – get down to business, the more the better! Concerning salt, utilize great quality ocean salt or Celtic salt to get helpful minerals and be sensible with it.

Solid fats like coconut oil, coconut drain and cream, ghee, margarine (correct, its generally fat so no issues with lactose), bow fat, jade oil, avocado oil, macadamia nut oil, fish oil, sesame oil and also from grass-bolster meats, rooster and fish.

Fixings like mustard, fish great, quality vinegars, for example, Fruit Juice with mother in it or matured Balsamic, low sugar tomato sauces and glue, olive oil mayonnaise, anchovies, olives, gherkins, escapades, salsas and prestos – are all fine, simply verify no dreadful chemicals and additives are included. Wheat free soy sauce, for example, Tamari and regularly determined clam sauce are alright occasionally however it's better to have a go at something like coconut amino.

For heating – nut dinners, flour of coconut, chestnut flour, sweet potato – use with some restraint as these fellows are either still high in sugars or may hold high measures of Omega-6 unsaturated fats. Keep this in mind seriously.

Prohibited Foods

Grains: particularly wheat and anything with gluten. White rice is the slightest unsafe of all grains and is frequently included to dishes events for assortment however its still high in starches and ought to be kept to "intermittent" utilization.

Vegetables: beans, lentils, chickpeas et cetera. Cashews are not vegetables! There are a few level headed discussions over whether a few vegetables are protected to devour with some restraint if arranged legitimately.

Refined sugars and carbs: bread, pasta, treats, white sugar, simulated sugar, high fructose syrup, soft drinks, and squeezes et cetera.

Dairy, particularly drain and low fat dairy and for those with harmed gut or gluten/lactose intolerances.

Prepared cooking oils and fats, for example, canola oil, soybean, some oilseed, flower oils, green and off course fresh vegetables and spreads made with such oils.

Desserts: Sugar is just about all fabricated and ought to be dodged in the primal diet. This methods is removing flavorful however ruinous desserts and sugars that are standard in the Standard American Diet. The general guideline here is: whether it has a huge amount of sugar – its most likely not primal. That said, here's a particular arrangement of desserts that are not on the primal diet nourishment rundown.

Chapter 3. Meal Plan for a Week

You may want to adopt Primal diet but still can't take any decision about daily meal or menu then you can follow this weekly plan for few weeks. This may be useful for you.

Monday

Breakfast: Eggs and vegetables, browned in coconut oil. One bit of tree grown foods.
Lunch: Chicken greens, with oil. Few barmy
Supper: Burgers (no bun), browned with vegetables and a few condiment.

Tuesday

Breakfast: Bacon and eggs, with a bit of tree grown foods.
Lunch: Leftover burgers from the prior night.
Supper: Salmon, browned and vegetables.

Wednesday

Breakfast: Meat with vegetables (scraps from night prior).

Lunch: Sandwich in a lettuce leaf, with meat and crisp vegetables.

Supper: Ground hamburger stir fry, with vegetables. A few berries.

Thursday

Breakfast: Eggs and a tree grown foods.

Lunch: Leftover stir fry from the prior night. Plenty nuts.

Supper: Fried pork and vegetables.

Friday

Breakfast: Eggs and vegetables, browned in coconut oil.

Lunch: Chicken greens with oil. Few barmy

Supper: Steak with vegetables and sweet potatoes.

Saturday

Breakfast: Bacon and eggs, with a bit of tree grown foods.

Lunch: Leftover steak and vegetables from the prior night.

Supper: Baked salmon with vegetables and avocado.

Sunday

Breakfast: Meat with vegetables (scraps from night prior).

Lunch: Sandwich in a lettuce leaf, with meat and new vegetables.

Supper: Grilled chicken with vegetables and salsa.

This is not a mandatory weekly plan you can add something new or the best way is to discuss with a nutritionist.

Chapter 4. Primal Recipes

Now-a- days lot recipes have been added with primal diet plan. Nutritionists and cocking specialists are inventing various recipes for primal diet. Some recipes have been stated in this book.

Bubbling Eggs for Deviled Eggs

Cooking the Eggs - Hard-bubbled eggs are simple and fast to get ready. Eggs in the shell ought to be cooked over high hotness simply until the water starts to Bubble then uprooted and left to remained until done. Never leave your eggs to bubble! In the event that eggs are bubbled for any period of time, the yolks will get hard on the other hand may turn an ugly greenish-light black. The methodology to full-evidence hard-bubbled eggs is a simple one. Basically put the eggs in a container spacious enough to hold them with icy water to blanket by no less than one inch. Next, over high hotness, warm the water and eggs until simply completely bubbling. When a full bubble is accomplished, expel the pan from the hotness, blanket hard and let them remained for 15 minutes. After the time has passed, spill off the boiling hot water and run cool water over the eggs to attain a quicker cooling. I let the frosty water run over the eggs for ten minutes furthermore add some ice to get them frosty quick. This not just stops the cooking process, however it likewise makes it simpler to peel the eggs. At that point I place them in the fridge for 60 prior minutes making the formula.

Shelling Hard-Cooked Eggs - Utilizing more seasoned eggs make this occupation a considerable measure simpler. Anyway you can escape with utilizing crisp eggs that you take after my strategy. Initially, you need to break the shells. The most straightforward approach to do this is to place all the eggs in a spacious pot again and shake them around. The tumult will split the shells pleasantly. At that point, to evacuate the shells, run each one egg under cool water and start to peel off bits of the shell. I generally begin at the substantial end; however it truly doesn't have any kind of effect.

Switzerland Chard Poker chips of Heated up Sesame

Ingredients:

Group rainbow Swiss chard

Bean stew sesame oil

Salt

Sesame seeds

First, divide leaves and also stalks from Swiss chard. Then you should wash and dry the clears out. It is critical to dry the leaves! In case the leaves are wet, then they can be saturated in the stove and not heat appropriately. Greens spinner works incredible for drying out the leaves, however you may need to provide for them an additional pat with paper towels simply to verify the majority of the water has been consumed.

Cover the Swiss chard leaves delicately with bean stew sesame oil. In the event that you are delicate to the hotness, don't hesitate to utilize consistent sesame oil. Sprinkle the leaves with sesame seeds and season with salt. Lay the Swiss chard forgets on top of a cooling rack in a solitary layer, considering some room between the takes off. Prepare in the preheated stove for 8-10 minutes, until the leaves are fresh.

Poultry Wings

Ingredients:

12 entire poultry parts

Oil of coconut in an amount of three ounces

1 little amount of garlic, compressed

1/4 glass warm sauce

one or two teaspoon fit salt

Put a six-quarter pan with a vapor wicker container and 1-creep of water in the base, over high hotness, blanket and heat to the point of boiling. Evacuate the tips of the wings and dispose of or put something aside for making stock. Utilizing kitchen shears, or a blade, divide the section at the joint. Put those into the steamer wicker compartment, spread, diminish the high temperature to medium and steam for 10 minutes. Oust the wings from the wicker compartment and meticulously pat dry. Put down those out on a chilling stand set in a half sheet skillet lined with paper cover and leave in the cooler for an hour. Supplant the paper towels with material paper. Broil on the center rack of the stove for 20 minutes. Turn the wings over and cook an additional 20 minutes or until meat is cooked through and the skin is brilliant tan. While the chicken is broiling, soften the coconut oil in a little bowl along with the garlic. Spill this alongside hot sauce and salt into a vessel substantial enough to hold the greater part of the chicken and mix to consolidate. Expel the wings from the stove and exchange to the dish and throw sauce and serve.

Meat Chomps

Ingredients:

 Sirloin meat- one pound (not including a large amount

cartilage) or precut meat tips

Genuine salt to taste

2 Tablespoons coconut oil

New ground dark pepper to taste

Trim off the substantial evident bit of fat that scuttle with the

meat area. Then, slash strips short of what one inch thick.

Pivot the meat and cut into little nibble estimated pieces. In

the event that you see any all the more huge pieces of fat,

cartilage then again long shiny layer, cut them off. Sprinkle

liberally with fit salt and newly ground pepper. Throw the

meat around a bit to completely layer with the seasonings.

Next, turn on your ventilation of overheating of the fan. Heat

the cooking pan over medium high to high hotness. As the

container warms, include something like 2 tablespoons

coconut oil to the skillet. Permit the oil to soften before you

include the meat. Put a percentage of the meat in the

container in a solitary layer. It ought to sizzle uproariously

when it hits the container - on the off chance that it doesn't,

the dish isn't hot enough. Don't mix or disturb the meat for

30-45 seconds. You need it to sizzle and tan on one side. Scoop the same number of steak chomps as you can with your spatula also flip them over. Rehash until all the meat is turned. Cook for an extra 30 to 45 seconds-sufficiently long to singe the outside of the meat yet NOT cook within. Uproot the meat to a clean plate. Add somewhat more oil to the skillet and rehash the cooking methodology with the following bunch almost as some time recently. Finally, when all the meat is pleasantly seared and uprooted to the plate, pour all that oil everywhere throughout the meat.

Bacon Wrapped Grill Shrimp

Ingredients:

16 extensive headless shrimp

8 cuts bacon

Grill flavoring, to taste

Clean and devein the shrimp, leaving the last segment of the tail. Wrap with 1/2 cut of bacon, securing with a toothpick. Make certain and utilize the substantial shrimp; the cooking time for the shrimp and the bacon is comparative. In the event that you do use mediums, you may need to precook the bacon a bit -over cooked shrimp are intense and rubbery, and a true sin! Line a jellyroll container with aluminum thwart and spot heating rack in skillet. Place the shrimp on the rack, and sprinkle with grill flavoring to taste; turn and sprinkle second side. Put aside for 15 to 20 minutes while the stove preheats. The bacon will turn from velvety white to sometime misty, and also the seasoned can absorb. Heat up stove to 450 degrees F (230 degrees C).

Prepare wrapped shrimp in preheated broiler for 10 to 15 minutes. The bacon should be fresh, and the shrimp pink and delicate. The rack keeps the shrimp from sitting in the emptying bacon fat.

Chapter 5. Benefits of Primal Diet for Human Body

The formal title Primal diet offering nourishment result from nuts, apples and oranges, berries and vegetables, the eating regimen additionally incorporates roots, fish and meat. An individual changes the calories expended every day to equivalent their lifestyle, so the busier they are, the more calories are required. This sounds extraordinary for a mountain man or cave dwellers, who were continually on the go to discover sustenance while abstaining from being a dinner for some other life structure. The danger of cardiovascular malady is one thing accepted to be brought down by this eating methodology. The end of bad fat by consuming characteristic, sound sustenance and getting more practice positively aides decrease the danger. Circulatory strain is come back to and stays at typical levels as opposed to raising and dropping at disturbing velocities. Evading dairy items, vegetables and entire grains sways adherents to consume eggs, shellfish and different things that the Stone Age man would have had the capacity to search. The skeletal framework is focused via convey abundance weight. Simply disposing of the additional tummy fat that hauls the spine flabby is leverage. Fitting weight helps enthusiastic wellbeing.

Those toting biscuit best over their pants know how pleasant it would be to attach their jeans without sucking in their gut first. Feeling better about the way we look is the consequence of a trim solid body.

Grown-up onset diabetes is a standout amongst the most perilous and exorbitant sicknesses in today's reality. Evading sugar, salt, fat (counting most oils) and soft drinks gives a healthier choice of sustenance and fluids for those at danger of this deadly ailment. The target of sustenance is survival and fulfillment. Incline proteins and plants convey those two objectives by giving protein, fiber and liquids. Holding glucose under control and lessening weight is an essential component in anticipating sort 2 diabetes. This adaptable eating methodology lets every individual conform it to their own particular tastes and needs. On the off chance that you hate fish, let it well enough alone for your nourishment plan. On the off chance that you love grapes, appreciate them. Overlooking the eating regimen and consuming greens finished with cheddar and ham on Friday evening does not make an individual a disgraceful miscreant. Consuming the right sustenance in the right amounts four days out of five will have a positive impact on your mental, passionate and physical being.

Conclusion

The primal diet, practically, and for most individuals, is going to comprise of a lot of crisp vegetables, great quality meats, fish and eggs, products of the soil, nuts and seeds. Individuals have varying perspectives about how strict one ought to be in watching a "legitimate" primal diet. At the end of the day it's going to be a matter of particular decision and, undoubtedly, accommodation. Some individuals are truly joyful to make primal adaptations of cutting edge sustenance, for example, pizza and cakes by making things like sweet potato brownies and cauliflower pizza base. Primal formulas like these will generally utilize current supplies, for example, sustenance processors, blenders and, obviously, a broiler - its barely an open fire in the mouth of a hole as indicated in all the best "stone age man" films! Objectors to this modernization have a tendency to demand that all sustenance ought to be bitten, as opposed to transformed - so smoothies have a tendency to be out - and for the most part a great deal less sweet than a large portion of us are utilized to.

Likely the best guidance is to attempt it for yourself and discover what works for you. The beginning stage for the primal diet, be that as it may, ought to dependably be to quit consuming grains, sugars, potatoes and vegetables, alongside all else that needs to be transformed before you can consume it. There is one more address, and that is whether you quit consuming dairy items. This level headed discussion between the primal diet (no dairy whatsoever) and primal consuming (some dairy permitted as long as you can endure it) seems to be, be that as it may, one that will need to sit tight for an alternate day!